HEALTH BETTER THAN SILVER AND GOLD

Written By

Verna E. MacKay

Health Better Than Silver And Gold

Dedication

This book is dedicated, to the King of Kings and Lord of Lords, Christ Jesus.

Samantha V. Small and Andrea M. Small.

"And as ye go, preach, saying, The kingdom of heaven is at hand. Heal the sick, cleanse the lepers, raise the dead, cast out devils: freely ye have received, freely give."

Matthew 10:7, 8.

Acknowledgment

All glory, praise and honor belongs to the Lord.
Thank you Lord for giving me the opportunity to serve
you and tell others of your wonderful love.
I acknowledge that with you all things are possible.

Cover designed by: Verna E. MacKay

Source of Authority

The Holy Bible.

God is the ultimate authority in everything.

Jesus is the "Alpha and Omega, the beginning and the ending."   Revelation 1:8

All Bible texts used in this book are from the King James Version.

Other books include the following

Jesus Christ God's Gift Of Love Our Hope Of Salvation.

The Prodigal Son

These are poems taken from the book Jesus Christ God's Gift Of Love Our Hope Of Salvation. Seven new poems have been added to this book.

Prayer And Praise From Earth To Heaven

God's Amazing Grace

Goats Sheep And Wolves

Waiting On The Lord

Website address

http://biblebased.weebly.com/

Email address: http//healthyliving635@gmail.com

Available in digital format on line.

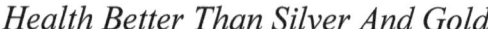

Health Better Than Silver And Gold

TABLE OF CONTENTS

Table of Contents

INTRODUCTION

Good health is better than all the silver and gold in the world. You may have a bank account filled with money, but if you are on your sick bed and you cannot get well, then the gold and silver is useless.

If you have lost your mind and have a bank account filled with millions of dollars, what good is it, if you cannot enjoy it?

Many things are needed to stay healthy, but until those things are implemented, and many companies seek to profit from your illness, then taking charge of your health and your body is of vital importance.

Chapter 1

Health Better Than Silver And Gold

"A little that a righteous man hath is better than the riches of many wicked." Psalm 37:16.

The bible records that there was a man, a beggar who could not walk, never walked a day in his life. Day after day, he was carried to the gate of the temple Beautiful to earn a living by begging money, from those who entered the temple. On this particular day, Peter and John were entering the temple to pray, and when they saw the man, they had compassion on him. Guided by the Holy Spirit they went over to where the man sat begging money, and told him to look at them.

The beggar that could not walk thought he was going to get money from Peter and John, but that day, he received something far more precious than silver and gold. Peter told the beggar to look at him, and told him he did not have any silver or gold to give him. Peter told the beggar, this is what I can give you, instead of money.

"Silver and gold have I none; but such as I have give I thee: In the name of Jesus Christ of Nazareth rise up and walk. And he took him by the right hand, and lifted him up: and immediately his feet and ankle bones received strength. And he leaping up stood, and walked, and entered with them into the temple, walking, and leaping, and praising God." Acts 3:6, 7, 8.

That day, this beggar who was lame from his mother's womb, met the true and living God, by way of Peter and John, received his health, something that was more precious than silver and gold, something that no silver and gold in the world could purchase. He received his health; no longer would he sit at the temple gate called Beautiful and earn a living day after day, depending on the kindness of strangers to support him. This man, this beggar ran, praised God, the one and only true God, Creator of heaven and earth, for what he had done for him.

For The Love Of Money

The bible tells us these words, "For we wrestle not against flesh and blood, but against principalities, against powers, against the rulers of the darkness of this world, against spiritual wickedness in high places." Ephesians 6:12.

Many times things are done to patients by doctors due to ignorance and the training they receive in medical school and many doctors seek to poison your body with prescription drugs, and profit from your illness, do not allow them to do so. Many good doctors think outside the box. They seek better natural alternatives for their patients.

Some doctors do the best for their patients, but there are many who is money driven. These unscrupulous, dishonest doctors, wicked doctors all belong in jail. Unfortunately, many of them are not caught, brought to justice, for the pain and suffering they inflected on their patients. One day, the Lord will deal with them and they will get exactly what they deserve. The Lord sees and he knows, and he will take care of the situation when the time is right.

Here is what the Lord says "Dearly beloved, avenge not yourselves, but rather give place unto wrath: for it is written, Vengeance is mine; I will repay, saith the Lord. Therefore if thine enemy hunger, feed him; if he thirst, give him drink: for in so doing thou shalt heap coals of fire on his head. Be not overcome of evil, but overcome evil with good." Romans 12:19, 20, 21.

There is a doctor who is will be going to prison for the rest of his life for giving unnecessary cancer treatment to his patients. Patients who did not have cancer told they have cancer, by this doctor and were discouraged from seeking another opinion from other doctors, were given harmful chemo and radiation. He did this for many years, destroying the life of those unfortunate patients who trusted him to take care of them. Had it not been for another doctor who saw what was going on and reported it, he would still be hurting people, all for the love of money.

This is not the first doctor who been charged, tried and put in prison for giving patients treatments they did not need, or given too much chemo, radiation, for illnesses they had, for the love of money.   It is important that you check out what the doctor tells you, by taking your health in your own hands, and seek a healthier approach.

Check out the doctor, to see if there are any complaints against him or her.   There are people who are masquerading themselves as doctors when they are not. Be very careful when you seek professional help, because you could be putting your life at risk. You can eat your way back to good health. Do not be so quick to believe everything your doctor tells you.

The bible says "The heart is deceitful above all things, and desperately wicked: who can know it? Jeremiah 17:9. Only the Lord knows the condition of the heart of man, and their motives.

Prescription Drugs

Some doctors write prescriptions drugs for their patients out of ignorance, because that is what they were trained to do. Since the creation of the internet, many people are coming to the realization that prescription drugs are not always the answer to the problem. Many people are taking charge of their health. They make a conscious decision to do what is necessary to stay healthy.

These prescription drugs come with horrible side effects, and while being advertised, the drug company mentions some of the side effects of the medication, including death. The actors you see in these advertisements are always smiling, having a wonderful time while being fed prescription drugs. Pain does not come with aging. Pain should not be managed and should not be a part of your everyday life. When you feel pain, your body is telling you it needs help. Constant inflammation of pain will destroy your body.

Find Out The Cause

If you are feeling pain, find out the cause of it and treat the cause, not the symptom. It is often said when an elderly person has aches and pains that it comes with old age, and is expected. That is sad, but doctors give pain relievers to treat the symptom, instead of treating the cause of the pain. If you come home one day, and find water on the floor, what are you going to do?

The first thing that you do is look to see where the water is coming from. You do not just take a mop and start mopping up the floor, because if you do, without finding out where the water is coming from, mopping up the floor is futile.

After finding out where the water is coming from, you shut off the source of the water, and then you mop up the floor. For example, the water maybe coming from the air conditioning unit, if that is the case, you turn off the unit, mop up the water and call a technician to fix the problem.

In this world, you will have only one body. Treat it with care, both on the inside as well as on the outside.

This is what the bible says "Know ye not that ye are the temple of God, and that the Spirit of God dwelleth in you? If any man defile the temple of God, him shall God destroy; for the temple of God is holy, which temple ye are." 1Corinthians 3:16, 17.

There are many health topics that are covered in this book, such as the benefits of good Nutrition, Exercise, Water, and Sunlight.

Exercise is a vital part of being healthy. Often times we do not realize the consequences of not exercising and even when we have the desire to exercise, we do not allow ourselves the opportunity to do so, maybe because of our busy schedules.

We live in a society, which does not afford us the opportunity to get the exercise we so desperately need, and our jobs may be one of the biggest obstacle. Companies realize that when an employee gets exercise during the day, they become more productive. Some companies have provided gyms for their employees because they see the positive results when exercise is added to the daily routine of their employees. This topic of exercise is covered in the exercise section.

<u>Remember</u>: in this life, you are given only one body and taking care of it is vital if you are to live a long, healthy and happy life.

God has given our bodies the means to heal itself. Drugs placed in the human body does more harm than good when natural remedies would be far better in helping the body heal itself. Natural remedies take a little longer to work, but they do work. They carry no nasty side effects like prescription drugs.

The information in this book is not intended to diagnose or treat any illnesses. Always check with your doctor or health practitioner and work with them in helping you become healthy.

Where Are The Nine

There is a spiritual aspect to good health. Neglecting the spiritual health is not good for anyone. The spiritual health is far better than the physical health, because when the person dies, and they die in the Lord will receive a new body that will never become sick.

The bible states that Jesus was on his way to Jerusalem, he traveled through Samaria and Galilee. When he was passing through an unnamed city, ten male lepers stood far away and cried out, asking Jesus to have mercy on them. Sometimes, we also cry out to Jesus to have mercy on us and help us, especially when we are sick. Lepers were not to mix with the general population, for the disease of leprosy is contagious.

Jesus had compassion on them and told them to go and show themselves to the priest. The priest had to examine them and test them to make sure they were cured of the disease. On their way to show themselves to the priest, they were healed. When one of them saw that they were cured of the leprosy, turned back to thank Jesus for healing him, and he glorified God, not with a soft voice, but shouts of joy. His shouts reached the throne room of heaven. He was grateful for what Jesus had done for him. He fell on his face at the feet of Jesus and worshiped him. The one who returned to give thanks to Jesus was a Samaritan, who the Jews hated.

The other nine lepers were also healed but they kept on walking, did not return to thank Jesus for healing them. They did not glorify God. This is what transpired, "And Jesus answering said, Were there not ten cleansed? but where are the nine?

There are not found that returned to give glory to God, save this stranger. And he said unto him, Arise, go thy way: thy faith hath made thee whole." Luke 17:17, 18, 19.

That day, the Samaritan leper received the greater healing, than the other nine ungrateful lepers did, he received both spiritual and physical health.

When Jesus does something for you, always remember to thank him, and give him praise. He takes notice when you are ungrateful. Develop an attitude of gratitude. Make a list of what the Lord has done for you, and thank him each day, worship him, it is part of the healing process, both spiritual and physical.

Be positive, it does wonders for the body and mind. Laugh, it is good medicine. Help others who need your help, if you are able to. Give a smile to those who visit you, they will come away amazed at your positive attitude. Do not complain about your situation, after a time people will avoid you, because all they hear from you, is how sick you are. Do not become despondent about your situation. Talk with the Lord he will never get tired when you bring your worries and your cares to him. He loves you very much. Take the time to study your bible, it is filled with words of encouragement, especially the Psalms.

Break The Tobacco Habit

Cigarette, chewing tobacco, cigars and other forms of tobacco is very dangerous to the body. The health principle is in the bible. All kinds of vices the devil uses to destroy the mind and body of his victims. These dangerous products sold to the population, destroy the lungs, the internal organs and will one day kill its victims, if they continue to smoke.

Cigarette smoking not only takes the life of those who use them, but also the lives of those exposed to them, who do not smoke. This is second hand smoke, and even the smell of the clothes of the smokers will claim the lives of non-smokers. The consequences of tobacco usage causes cancer, breathing problems, inflammation of the lungs and other health related diseases.

Telling a smoker that cigarette smoking is bad for them is futile, because they know what the dangers are. If you sincerely desire to stop the destruction of your body by using harmful drugs and other substances, the Lord will help you. Lemon or lime is a good way to help you with nicotine dependency. Suck on a lemon or lime when you feel the urge to smoke. Drink lemon or lime water first thing in the morning before a meal, to help to clean up the blood stream. Do not believe the lies of the enemy Satan, because he wants to keep you in prison, by pacing harmful drugs in your body. You can overcome the addiction by asking the Lord for help to break the nicotine habit. This is best thing to do. Jesus is standing by, ready and willing to help you.

The Spiritual Aspect Of Health

"And it came to pass, as Jesus sat at meat in the house, behold, many publicans and sinners came and sat down with him and his disciples. And when the Pharisees saw it, they said unto his disciples, Why eateth your Master with publicans and sinners? But when Jesus heard that, he said unto them, They that be whole need not a physician, but they that are sick." Matthew 9:10, 11, 12.

When Jesus, God's only Son was on earth in human form, he healed all manner of sicknesses. He healed the lame, the blind, raised the dead, and forgave sins.

This aspect of healing was important, but the spiritual health is of vital importance. Jesus never neglected to let the ones who were physically sick know that he forgiven them of their sins.

You can achieve healing for your disease, but it is God how heals you, not the drugs that you take, even if you may not recognize the God of the universe. He does not discriminate; he sends the rain on the believers and those who do not believe on him, or accepts him as their Lord and Savior. He sends the sunshine and it shines on the believers as well as on the unbelievers. He loves everyone, the sinners as well as the righteous.

Sick Unto Death

King Hezekiah sick and he were going to die. When the Lord informed him that he was going to die, did not take the news of his impending death very well. If you were going to die and the Lord told you, you might do what King Hezekiah did. He turned his face toward the wall and cried bitterly.

The Lord sent his servant Isaiah the prophet to tell King Hezekiah to take a lump of figs, make a plaster and put it on the boil and this would heal him. The Lord added fifteen more years to the king's life. See 2 Kings 20:6.

King Hezekiah was very rich, but all the silver and gold he had could give him back his health. It could not save his life, only the Lord could, by healing his disease.

Go And Sin No More

There was a man by the water waiting to be placed in the water, for it was said that at a certain time, an angel came and troubled the water. The person who got into the water first was healed. This man was sick of thirty-eight years. It seemed that Jesus debatably sought out this man, knowing his condition, and asked him if he wanted to be healed.

Of course, the man wanted healing, but what a strange question for Jesus to ask. The man told Jesus that he had no one to put him into the water when the angel troubled it. Jesus told him to take up his bed and go his way; Jesus healed him from his illness.

It seemed that this man's illness was due to some sin he committed which caused him to become sick. Later on Jesus found him and this is what Jesus said to him. "Afterward Jesus findeth him in the temple, and said unto him, Behold, thou art made whole: sin no more, lest a worse thing come unto thee." John 5:14.

Sometimes the illness we have was brought on us because we violate Gods health laws, and we suffer the consequences of that sin. If after the Lord heals you, and you continue with the same sin, the same habit that brought on the illness, you will become sick again. This time the sickness may be worse than the sickness before, and will lead to death.

You know you have an addiction to gambling, and the Lord delivered you from it, do not go to places where they gamble, or hang around people who gamble. If you do, you will find yourself in the same or worse situation than you did before. Whatever the habit is stay away from places and people who will entice into the same sin. *Health comes in various forms, financial, spiritual, mental, and physical.*

Getting Your Attention

The Lord wants desperately to save the world. He suffered and died for you. He arose from the grave and is now in heaven making intersession for you to the Father.

God will do everything he can to save you. He will go through every means possible to save your life, so you can live with him forever throughout the ceaseless ages.

After trying to get your attention and you refuse to listen to his voice, will allow certain things to happen to you so he can save you. It may be an illness, an accident, prison, and so forth. Now you will have to listen because you have nowhere else to go. He will reason with you, he will agonize with you, and finally you will begin to see and listen to his voice as he speaks to you.

Many people spend their time running away from the Lord, but the Lord will never get tired of seeking the lost, and when that lost person finally listens, accepts

Jesus as their personal Savior, all of heaven rejoices. Now you see that the spiritually sick person is healed from his spiritual condition. They may also be healed from their physical illness. If you truly and sincerely desire to be healed, you must completely depend on the Lord. He is the one who heals you, not the drugs you take. What an amazing and awesome God.

Chapter 2

Nutrition And You

Nutrition is a vital part of being healthy. There are laws of health, which God gave us written in his holy book, the bible. Proper nutrition is a vital part of being healthy and staying healthy. When you break any of the laws you will suffer the negative consequences, in other words you become sick. The Lord has not left us in darkness regarding the things we are to put in our bodies, and the things we should leave out. These rules still apply today, they are not just for the children of Israel, but for this whole world. Here are some of the dietary laws the Lord gave. Violate the health principles you will get sick with various kinds of illnesses, and wonder why you are sick, suffering, and dying.

"And the LORD spake unto Moses and to Aaron, saying unto them, These are the beasts which ye shall eat Whatsoever parteth the hoof, and is clovenfooted, and cheweth the cud, among the beasts, that shall ye eat. These shall ye not eat of them that chew the cud, or of them that divide the hoof: And the hare, because he cheweth the cud, but divideth not the hoof; he is unclean unto you. And the swine, though he divide the hoof, and be clovenfooted, yet he cheweth not the cud; he is unclean to you.

These shall ye eat of all that are in the waters: whatsoever hath fins and scales in the waters, in the seas, and in the rivers, them shall ye eat. And all that have not fins and scales in the seas, and in the rivers, of all that move in the waters, and of any living thing which is in the waters, Whatsoever hath no fins nor scales in the waters." See the book of Leviticus chapter 11.

The devil has sought to destroy the human race through appetite. Adam and Eve were tempted to eat from the tree God told them not to eat from, and by listening to the lies from the enemy, ate and plunged the world into sin.

During the temptation of Jesus by the devil after fasting for forty days, the devil knowing how hungry Jesus was, told him to turn the stones into bread.

Jesus met him with scripture by not allowing himself to give into the temptation of appetite. Too many times the devil tempts you to put into your body the things that will destroy your body. The Lord wants you to be healthy because he loves and cares for you.

Given a chance, man will eat just about anything that they can get into their mouth, and into their stomach. Poor nutrition affects the animals as well because the manufacturers of the dog food, cat food and other domesticated animals are fed animal byproducts and chemicals in their food that destroy their bodies. The dogs have the flu, the fish in the ocean and in the rivers by known and unknown diseases, the chicken has the bird flu and at the time this book was written, millions of chicken had to be destroyed due to the bird flu.

Some human beings have lost their minds, they are not healthy, and many kept alive with the use of harmful drugs that destroy both body and mind. Our foods are manufactured in labs, altered, and experimented on, and when eaten brings diseases on those who unknowingly purchase these foods.

Harmful chemicals are added to the foods made by manufacturing companies, which affects the health of the consumers.

Some of these harmful things found in your food are hydrogenated oil, partially hydrogenated oils, BHT, bromide, saturated fats, canola oil, Tran's fat and other harmful chemicals too numerous to list.

Fluoride which is a poison is added to the water supply, is in our toothpaste, and the public is getting these poisons in their system, causing many illnesses. Some of the foods the public eat such as cabbage, corn, wheat, and other foods are experimented on in a lab injected with human and animal DNA. Harmful pesticides have been added to the foods you eat. Antibiotics given to the animals passed on to you when you eat the flesh of these animals.

Daniel and his three friends, Sadrach, Meshach and Abednego (Hananiah, Mishael, and Azariah their real names) when taken from their homes in Jerusalem and brought into the king's place refused to eat the food provided for them by the king. They had been trained from home what they should and should not eat.

Imagine how brave these young men were, who depended on their God for everything they needed, and trusted in him, obeyed him by rejecting the destructive food they were required to eat. They made up their minds not to be defiled by what the king was serving, but to obey the commands of the Lord.

This is what they requested, "Prove thy servants, I beseech thee, ten days; and let them give us pulse to eat, and water to drink. Then let our countenances be looked upon before thee, and the countenance of the children that eat of the portion of the king's meat: and as thou seest, deal with thy servants. So he consented to them in this matter, and proved them ten days." Daniel 1:12, 13 and 14.

What was the result after eating this diet of pulse (a variety of beans and peas including lentils) and drinking water for ten days? God blessed them tremendously for obeying his health statutes and his commands. The result was wonderful. The bible state that "And at the end of ten days their countenances appeared fairer and fatter in flesh than all the children which did eat the portion of the king's meat." Daniel 1:15. When these young men brought before the king spoke with them, they found to be full of knowledge and wiser than all the other young men were.

Many of you are health conscious, and desire to become healthy, and to stay healthy by eating as nutritionally as you possibly can. You are living in an environment, a world where what you eat, even when being health conscious, due to man's greed for money, will somehow affect your health. Do the best that you can, and ask the Lord to help you.

The bible states, "And the LORD will take away from thee all sickness, and will put none of the evil diseases of Egypt, which thou knowest, upon thee; but will lay them upon all them that hate thee." Deuteronomy 7:15

"And said, If thou wilt diligently hearken to the voice of the LORD thy God, and wilt do that which is right in his sight, and wilt give ear to his commandments, and keep all his statutes, I will put none of these diseases upon thee, which I have brought upon the Egyptians: for I am the LORD that healeth thee." Exodus 15:26.

Today, the bodies of the Egyptians are exhumed and examined by scientists to find out the causes of their death. They were dying of many kinds of illness such as heart attacks, high blood pressure, high cholesterol levels, and other diseases.

Poor nutrition breaks down the immune system and leaves the body susceptible to many illnesses. Poor nutrition is very bad for the body, and when the diet is lacking in nutrients, such as vitamins and minerals, the whole body cannot function properly. Put only what is healthy in your body, and your body will thank you and pay you back with good health.

"Bless the LORD, O my soul: and all that is within me, bless his holy name.

Bless the LORD, O my soul, and forget not all his benefits:

Who forgiveth all thine iniquities; who healeth all thy diseases;

Who redeemeth thy life from destruction; who crowneth thee with lovingkindness and tender mercies; Who satisfieth thy mouth with good things; so that thy youth is renewed like the eagle's."

Psalm 103:1, 2, 3, , 5.

Poor Diets Are Dangerous To Your Health

Diets that are lacking in nutrients are the cause a vast array of illnesses in the human body. If our bodies are not getting the nutrients that it needs to function properly, after a while, it is going to break down and become diseased.

When God made us, he gave us a manual. This manual includes good dietary habits, principles designed to teach us how to take care of our bodies and the proper nutrients we should put into our bodies.

When you decide to incorporate good nutrition as part of your lifestyle, you will become healthy. Poor nutrition and foods void of nutritional value will destroy the human body.

When you purchase a vehicle, that vehicle comes with a manual that tells you how to take care of it. The manufacturer of the vehicle tells you to put gasoline in the vehicles gas tank. What would happen if you disobeyed the manufacturer of the vehicle and put in things such as water, oil and sand in the vehicles gas tank? The vehicle would break down and stop functioning and if the damage is very bad, the auto mechanic may not be able to fix the vehicle. Well, that can and often times happen to the human body that God gave us. Sometimes the damage due to poor nutrition is so bad the doctors cannot help you, they do not get to the cause of the problem, and they are busy writing prescription, which they give you to take, when all you needed was proper nutrients and a healthy lifestyle.

A person dies from not getting proper nutrients in the body. The results of an improper diet (poor nutrition) causes a person get high blood pressure, diabetes, heart disease, kidney disease, all forms or cancer, gallstones, gallbladder infections, insomnia, obesity, constipation, and the list goes on, and on, and on.

Some people know that the cause of their illnesses is due to their diet, but continue to eat the things they know they should not eat. The eating of swine (pigs) flesh is not to be eaten, they are unclean and they are the cause of many illness. Creatures in the sea that has no fins or scales should not be eaten. They were created by God to clean the bodies of water that God created.

People pray to the Lord asking for healing and wonder why the Lord does not answer their prayers. Why should the Lord heal them when they refuse to change their bad eating habits, and continue their poor lifestyle? There are many people who know that they should give up certain foods, and chose a more healthy lifestyle instead, refuses to make the necessary changes, even when their bodies are dying from these diseases, would rather die eating what they love, and go to an early grave.

They stop their ears, close their eyes and say that you are going to die of something. Why die a painful miserable death that could have been avoided, by changing the diet, eating nutritious food and live many years longer. How very sad.

What The Bible Says About Health

God said, "Behold, I have given you every herb bearing seed, which is upon the face of the earth, and every tree, in the which is the fruit of a tree yielding seed, to you it shall be for meat." Genesis 1:29.

Our original diet in the beginning was herb, seeds (nuts and grains) and fruits free to us from the hands of God. This was a complete original diet packed with nutrients to supply the body with proper nutrition designed to keep us healthy.

After man sinned, for added nutrition God added vegetables to our diet. Vegetables have chlorophyll, which makes the plant green. Chlorophyll is similar (almost identical) to the blood that we have running through our veins, so each time we eat vegetables we are actually giving ourselves a blood transfusion.

The herbs, nuts, grains and fruits in its natural state have many nutrients that the body needs. The seeds and nuts when used in its natural state will supply the body with proper nutrition. The nuts and seeds should not be roasted and should be free of salt. These nuts when grounded up can be used in a variety of ways that will be of benefit to the body. They can be used to make bread, shakes, toppings, milk, cheese, cheese sauce, salad dressing, added to salads, eaten in their natural state, and very nourishing to the body.

Foods To Avoid And Healthy Alternatives

Some foods stripped of their nutrients and a few vitamins added back to them; do not supply the full nutritional value to the food. Some of the foods that have been stripped of its nutritional value are brown rice, cornmeal, and whole-wheat flour.

White rice and white flour is very bad for the human body and it is void of nutrients, causes constipation and many other health related problems. White sugar should be classified as a drug, it provides no nutritional value, and should never be put in the body because it is poisonous to the system, which causes a wide range of diseases. Sugar in any form is bad for the human body including brown sugar. In fact, some manufacturers actually take the white sugar, cover it with molasses, and package it as brown sugar, which is void of nutrients.

Healthy substitute for sugar would be pure honey, stevia and maple syrup. Unsulphured black strap molasses is nutritionally very good because it contains a vast amount of nutrients such as calcium, iron, carbohydrate, potassium, manganese and magnesium. In fact, blackstrap molasses because of its high iron content is used to treat anemia.

The bible tells states we are not to eat the blood or the fat of these animals. If the animal is sick, and you eat the blood and the fat, you will become sick. The bible states "The life of the flesh is in the blood: No soul of you shall eat blood, neither shall any stranger that sojourneth among you eat blood." Leviticus 17: 11, 12. You may say that was Old Testament, but also in the New Testament, the Apostle Paul says "abstain from blood, and from things strangled." Acts 15:29.

People today eat their meat with blood in it; they do not realize that they are brining diseases upon themselves. When they come down with things such as cancer, especially colon cancer, they wonder why they are sick. Poor food choices made today, will affect your health in a negative way in the years to come. When the body is abused, it remembers and will pay you back for all the years of torture you inflected on it.

Sodas And Caffeine – Bad For Your Health

Caffeine is a drug, which provides no nutrients to the body, found in many products such as sodas, sports drinks, tea, coffee, shakes, and chocolate. Even some caffeine free products have a small amount of caffeine in it.

Caffeine destroys the brain cells, brain tissues, produces insomnia, it triggers stress hormones, is addictive and these are just a few of the many bad side effects it has on the body. So called energy drinks contains no nutrients and should be avoided like the plague. They contain a vast amount of caffeine and other ingredients, which is very bad for your health. Sports drinks (devoid of nutrients), and vitamin water should be avoided because they contain high volume of sugar and other ingredients that are not good for the body.

Soda is loaded with sugar and it takes a lot of water to dilute one can of soda and its void of nutrients, in other words, it has no nutritional value. Soda leaches the calcium and magnesium from the bones leading to brittle bones which eventually leads to osteoporosis, obesity, tooth decay, heart disease, neurological disorders, nutritional deficiencies just to name a few and contains large amounts of caffeine.

Dumping The Excess Baggage

Excessive oils and fats in the system clog the arteries and leads to heart attack, especially animal fats. We should avoid food additives, which supplies no nutritional value. Excessive amounts of sugar should not be consumed, even the good ones such as honey, maple syrup and other sugars. All things that we do should be done in moderation. We should be temperate in all things.

Artificial sweeteners should not be placed in the human body because it destroys the body and is void of nutrients. Excessive salt leads to water retention, high blood pressure and other health related problems. Two of the best types of salt are Celtic Sea Salt and Himalayan Salt. These salts are unrefined and contain balanced minerals, and trace elements such as calcium, magnesium, potassium, copper and iron.

Poor nutritional choice such as refined foods should be never be put in the body, because they destroy the body and have no nutrients in them. Some of these are white flour products, refined cornmeal products, sugar, oils and fats.

The use of baking soda and baking power is very harmful to the body including aluminum free baking powder, these two causes inflammation of the stomach, which poisons the system. When baking soda is placed in water it expands and bubbles, and so it does in our bodies.

God intended for the human race to be healthy with the use of proper nutrition. The use of vinegar or anything containing vinegar should be avoided since it is bad for the stomach and contains no nutrients. Vinegar used for cleaning, acts as an embalmer within the system and should not be placed in the body. Vinegar destroys the lining of the stomach, which robs the body of nutrients. Use lemon or lime juice as a substitute for vinegar.

The use of ice cream should be avoided and is void of proper nutrients. When sugar and milk are combined together, it turns to alcohol in the stomach. If you must eat ice cream, try the vegetarian one, which found at health food stores. Any ice-cold beverages including water should be avoided because it destroys the lining of the stomach. Spicy foods should be avoided for the same reason.

On the cross, Jesus was thirsty, they gave him vinegar to drink and he refused to drink it when he tasted it and found out it was vinegar. Matthew 27:34.

Eating Healthy Meals

Too much food and too much of a variety of foods that are eaten at one meal is not good. This is very bad for the system. At each meal, we should limit the variety of foods we eat. For example, we should eat no more than three different kinds of fruit at one meal.

We should space our meals at least five hours apart. If breakfast, which is the main meal of the day, is eaten at 7:00 a.m. then lunch should be eaten five hours later giving our digestive system a chance to digest the earlier meal and to rest. If we eat our meal at 7:00 a.m. then another meal, again at 8:00 a.m., we disrupt the digestive process, when new food is added to the system; the digestion process starts all over again. Food in the system begins to rot causes fermentation in the body, which is very bad.

In between meals, we should drink plenty of good quality water. If it is at all possible, try to eat meals each day at the same time. You may also drink natural fruit juices that have some fiber in it (not sugary refined fruit juice) between meals. Fresh vegetables and fruits juiced and consumed at the time it is juiced is very healthy for the body. Do not drink a glass full of juiced vegetables and fruits because it is too much.

How many carrots would you eat at one sitting, ask yourself this question. How many fruits would you consume at the same time? You would not eat that many, so when you juice, so consider these questions which will give you a guideline when drinking freshly juiced fruits and vegetables. Your mouth and your stomach is a juice extractor. The body absorbs the juice and the fiber is used to clean the colon and passed through the system when you use the bathroom. You should not strain to have a bowel movement when you use the bathroom if you are getting fiber in your diet.

You should never eat and drink with your meals. This causes health problems later on.

Number Of Meals To Eat Each Day

If it is at all possible, (especially if you are trying to lose weight) eat only two meals per day. The morning meal, which is breakfast, and afternoon meal, which is lunch, should be heavy. The evening meal should be very light consisting of fruits and bread and or soup is a better meal option.

(Note: If your profession requires heavy lifting and manual labor such as construction, then you will require more food at the end of the day.). Eat according to the type of work you do at any given meal but do not over eat. Over eating puts a burden on the digestive system.

It is said that we should eat like a king in the mornings, a prince at lunch and a pauper at night. The evening meals should be eaten three hours or more before going to bed. This allows your digestive system rest while you sleep.

Dangers Of Eating And Drinking With Your Meals

When you eat and drink with your meals you dilute the gastric juices (stomach acids) needed to digest your meals and you destroy your digestive system. Look at it this way, what happens when you throw water on a fire? The fire goes out. The same with your gastric juices, and eating and drinking with your meals over a period of years you find yourself popping antacids (which does not solve the problem but create more problems for the system) you end up with various kinds of stomach problems such as, H-pylori, acid reflux, low stomach acids and heartburn.

Drinking should be done half-hour before a meal and one and a half to two hours after a meal. When you chew our food, you should chew until it is liquefied, because digestion begins in the mouth. By the time the food reaches our stomach, it should be partially digested, thereby giving your digestive system less work to do.

The Lord Want You To Be Healthy

"The thief cometh not, but for to steal, and to kill, and to destroy: I am come that they might have life, and that they might have it more abundantly." John 10:10.

The devil is the thief; he wants you to be sick so you will not hear the voice of the Lord when he speaks to you. The devil seeks to destroy you, and solicits your help in destroying yourself. Why should you pay manufacturers to destroy your own body with the things they call food, that is not good for human consumption. They pack their products full of harmful chemicals; hide them under fancy names, so you will not detect their deceit, knowing these foods will destroy your health.

This is what the Lord says, "But they that will be rich fall into temptation and a snare, and into many foolish and hurtful lusts, which drown men in destruction and perdition.

For the love of money is the root of all evil: which while some coveted after, they have erred from the faith, and pierced themselves through with many sorrows.

But thou, O man of God, flee these things; and follow after righteousness, godliness, faith, love, patience, meekness." 1Timothy 6:9, 10, 11.

The Lord wants you to be healthy. He does not want you to be sick. The bible states "Beloved, I wish above all things that thou mayest prosper and be in health, even as thy soul prospereth." 3 John 1:2.

It is very important that you eat nourishing meals each day that is full of nutrition, a meal consisting of nuts, grains, fruits, vegetables and plenty of good quality water. If you decided to make a change to a healthier lifestyle regarding your nutritional intake, try to do it gradually so that you do not become overwhelmed.

Some people can make the nutritional changes faster than some people can. A plant-based diet is the best because it is nutritious. For vegan recipes do a search on the internet and you will find many good nutritional recipes, which will give you a start to a healthier and happier life, and these recipes will show you how to make burgers and meat loaf substitute using nuts and grains.

Use brown rice, which is more nutritional instead of white rice, and use Non GMO whole-wheat, soy flour, brown rice flour and oatmeal flour instead of white flour, and lemon juice instead of vinegar.

Many other good nutritional foods can be added to your diet such as red rice, wild rice, barley and quinoa. The use of garlic is very good, a variety of onions, variety of bell peppers, lettuce, non GMO cabbage, okra, beans, carrots, tomatoes, and so much more. God has given the human race a variety of good food to eat. The food God has given to the human race is full of vitamins and minerals, which helps to rebuild the body each day, and to keep the mind healthy.

After Adam and Eve were driven from the Garden of Eden, they had to work to keep the body and mind in shape, which was hard work. This is what the Lord said and did according to the bible, " And unto Adam he said, Because thou hast hearkened unto the voice of thy wife, and hast eaten of the tree, of which I commanded thee, saying, Thou shalt not eat of it: cursed is the ground for thy sake; in sorrow shalt thou eat of it all the days of thy life; Thorns also and thistles shall it bring forth to thee; and thou shalt eat the herb of the field;" Genesis 3:17, 18. When the bible speaks about it, the Lord is speaking about the earth.

Alcohol – Dangerous To Your Health

Another of Satan's deception is the use of alcohol. The bible is very clear when it comes to the use of alcohol. The Lord wants you to stay away from it, because it is dangerous to the body. It has destroyed families, leave them in poverty, and turn a home into hell on earth. Children are abused, wives and it goes for husbands are abused, health damaged including the mind.

The devils intension is to deceive you into thinking that alcohol is good for you, so he gets other humans help in saying that it is good to drink alcoholic beverages because it has health benefits. You can get the same benefits from drinking grape juice without the alcohol. If you mind is clogged and destroyed by alcohol, you cannot hear the voice of the Holy Spirit when the Lords bids you come to him, surrender your life to him, because he loves you, and wants you to be healthy. Without the Lord in your life, Satan will seek to destroy you by lying to you, about the dangers of alcohol.

Alcohol poisons the body, the internal organs, the blood, the mind, and the list of evils caused by this demon is quite extensive. This bible says "Wine is a mocker, strong drink is raging: and whosoever is deceived thereby is not wise." Proverbs 20:1.

In the bible the wisest man that ever lived King Solomon, says this about alcohol, "Who hath woe? who hath sorrow? who hath contentions? who hath babbling? who hath wounds without cause? who hath redness of eyes? They that tarry long at the wine; they that go to seek mixed wine. Look not thou upon the wine when it is red, when it giveth his colour in the cup, when it moveth itself aright. At the last it biteth like a serpent, and stingeth like an adder." Proverbs 23:29 – 32.

Chapter 3

Exercise What Is So Good About It?

So what is so good about exercise? Answer: Getting regular physical exercise is very important to the body and has many health benefits. When you exercise it puts you in a very good mood, it eases depression and in some cases will eliminates it.

Exercise adds years to your life, it is very good for the heart; it helps you to lose weight and keep it under control. Exercise builds muscle, reduces the chances of getting certain types of cancer such as colon and breast, reduces high blood pressure and in some cases eliminates it.

Exercise is beneficial for those who are diabetic; exercise reduces bad cholesterol level and increases the good cholesterol level, exercise lessens the possibility of strokes, has a positive effect on the thyroid glands, stimulates bone growth, reduces the risk of osteoporosis, and sometimes eliminates it all together.　Exercise helps to remove toxins from the body through the eliminating organs.

How Are Toxins Eliminated From The Body Through Exercise?

The skin is the largest organ and when you exercise you perspire, when you perspire you eliminate toxins from your body. You eliminate toxins through the kidney when you urinate so when you exercise you help your internal organs to eliminate toxins from your body. You eliminate toxins through the salivary glands, lymph nodes and the colon. These are just some of the example of how toxins are eliminated from your body through exercise.

Running And Jogging Good Forms Of Exercise?

The problem with jogging and running as a form of exercise is that it puts a lot of weight and strain on the joints, which causes a lot of wear and tear. For example, a person's weight is 150 pounds, 200 pounds and even less and they run and jog on a regular basis as a form of exercise, after a number of years or even less time, they begin to develop pain in the joints of the knees and eventually this leads to knee surgery intended to correct the problem.

Pay close attention to the advertisements on the TV, sports magazines, internet and other places of advertisement. You find advertisements from doctors, hospitals regarding knee replacements. The fluids between the joints are depleted and other injuries have occurred. Bone is now rubbing on bone causing pain and suffering. Keep your joints healthy, and you will not need to have these problems as you age.

Trying To Lose Weight

The best form of exercise is walking at a fast pace outdoors. This gives the body a total work out including getting the heart rate up which is very important in maintaining good health, in other words it gives you a good cardiovascular workout. Exercising outdoors gets fresh air in your lungs, which is beneficial to the body.

Working out at the gym is a good form of exercise. Using the machines to help to strengthen your legs, and build muscle, can be of benefit to you. Using the treadmill is good but exercising without a treadmill is far better.

With the treadmill, even though you are walking you are not getting all the benefits of the sunshine and the fresh air to fill your lungs as you do with walking. With the treadmill as a form of exercise, you are not getting a total body workout as you do with walking outdoors and walking is free, no monthly or yearly fees to pay. If you live near a beach, use it as an exercise fitness tool, take advantage of it and get that clean air into your lungs. Take deep breaths, breathe in through your nostrils and breathe out through your mouth, this sends oxygen to the brain. Now if you are not used to getting oxygen to the brain, you may want to sit while you are breathing in and out because it will make you dizzy, and getting oxygen to the brain is very important for good brain health.

Walking in the park is good way to exercise and some parks have exercise trails with exercise instructions or anywhere you can find to walk that suites your needs. If you are trying to lose weight, the best form of exercise is walking. You can even walk in the house if it is a rainy day and still get the benefits of exercise. Be creative and have fun while you exercise.

If you are trying to lose weight, you should walk for a minimum of one hour per day without breaks in between. Exercising for thirty minutes per day outside will cause your respiratory rate and pulse rate to go up or rise.

If you are not exercising to lose weight but just to stay fit then you can break up your exercise in fifteen minutes, ten minutes intervals to add up to the total time needed. In other words, you do not have to exercise for one hour straight or for thirty minutes straight if you are not able to and still get the benefits of a good workout.

When you go to the store, instead of parking close to the entrance, park farther away and walk. This is a good way of getting some exercise. Have small children who love to stand or sit on your feet. Use them as weights to help you keep in shape. Swing the up and down on your feet, they enjoy it and so will you.

Other Good Forms Of Exercise

Another good exercise to do is bicycling and cycling. Now if you are a male, you may not want to do this too often in order to protect the prostrate.

Before starting, an exercise program check with your doctor and let him or her know what you starting an exercise program. If you are having a lot of health issue, start slow and gradually increase your exercise rate. Gardening is another good form of exercise. Do you know that house cleaning is another form of exercise, mopping, dusting, vacuuming, but in addition to that, you need to walk especially if you are trying to get lose weight. Before starting to exercise, be sure to do some stretching exercises first.

You can also do some jumping jacks; if you are starting for the first time then do about ten then as you continue increase the number according to your ability.

Try some weight bearing exercise to keep the bones in shape and make them strong, exercise such as lifting weights is good. Start out with small weights first such as 1.5 pounds for each hand and ankle then increase as your arms and legs get stronger, when using weights do not walk with ankle weights on your ankle. Golfing is another good form of exercise, volleyball, basketball, tennis, racquetball and other sports are good forms of exercise.

Jumping Jacks Exercise Instructions

Begin with your hands at your side and your feet together, spread your legs apart and raise your arms over your head in single jumping motion. Return arms and legs together and continue.

No, lifting the remote control to change the channel on the TV or DVR is not a form of exercise and neither is lifting the fork and spoon to your mouth. Remember, have fun while you are exercising. Having a buddy system including some of your friends, your spouse, your children and your relatives, have them join you in your exercise quest for good health. This will help to motivate each of you and it is a win, win situation for all involved.

Cut down on the amount of time that you spend in front of the idiot box, put the remote control down, get outside and exercise. It will benefit you greatly. Remember, the Lord wants you to be healthy.

Chapter 4

Water Does A Body Good

Water is very important to the body because it flushes toxins out of your system. Our bodies are made up of approximately 60 to 80 percent water depending what our ages are.

When we are born, our body is mostly water and as we age that percentage of water becomes less depending on whether you are a male or female. The point being, you need to drink a lot of water per day to help your body remove waste and to quench your thirsts.

We can go a little over a month without eating but only approximately three days without water. You should drink approximately eight to twelve glasses of water per day depending on your size and your age. A small child will not require as much water as an adult.

If you are working outside your body will require more water, than someone who works indoors at a desk each day. Drink water according to the occupation that you do. When the time is cold make sure you get plenty of water to drink, even though you may not want to. Do not allow the change of seasons to dictate the amount of water you drink.

How Can You Tell If You Are Getting Enough Water To Drink?

 A good way of telling if you are getting enough water is to look at your urine. If your urine is not clear then you are not getting enough water and you need to drink more water.

Take into consideration that if you are taking vitamin supplements or medication your urine will reflect the color of the supplements or medication but you should be able to tell the difference.

Water Should Not Be Ice Cold

Water should be tepid or at room temperature when
you drink it. Ice-cold water cramps the system and in
order for the body to utilize the water and to refresh
your cells it (the body) has to heat the water, bring it
down to the temperature of the body before it
becomes available to the body to use.   This applies to
other fluids also.

Water - Drinking

Water should be filtered or purified, distilled or from a clean spring. You can, get a ten-stage water filter, or a better filter, which can be purchased at a health food store, or on line. These water filters last up to a year or more depending on the amount of water that is used. When taking a shower the water should not be hot but tepid. Remember that everything should be done in moderation.

Do not drink too much or too little water. Drinking too much water can drown the system causing health issues including flushing out your electrolytes and too much water puts too much strain on the kidneys. In actuality by drinking too much water, you are drowning your internal organs and stressing them out.

Drinking too much water can affect your brain causing the cells to swell and you may experience a headache, in fact, you could die from drinking too much water in a short period.

Drinking too little water can cause you to have a stroke, and you will lose brain cells. By the time you feel thirsty you have already lost several brain cells so do not wait until you feel thirst to drink water. A feeling of being thirsty tells you that you are dehydrated. Drink plenty of water when you are outdoors working, exercising and when the time is hot.

The elderly should be given water to drink throughout the day, even if they tell you they do not feel thirsty. As the body ages the thirst, mechanism does not function as it should.

If you have a headache, ask yourself this question: "Did I get enough water to drink today?" If the answer is no then your headache is most likely caused from not getting enough water to drink. Sometimes when you feel hungry, you may be thirsty and not hungry especially if we ate a short time ago. Sometimes we confuse thirst with hunger. Remember that pure clean clear water is very important to your body so drink, be healthy and happy.

The bible states "And Moses lifted up his hand and struck the rock with his staff twice, and water came out abundantly, and the congregation drank, and their livestock." Numbers 20:11.

Showering And Bathing

Try not to spend too much time in the shower or soaking in the bath, unless you have a filter on the faucets, or a whole house water filter.

The water in the pipe has too much chlorine, fluoride and bromide. These chemicals are harmful to the body. Look at the toothpaste box and you will see a warning on it, telling you to call a poison control center, if you accidently get too much in your system.

Water Therapy And Salt Glow Bath

There are many uses for water. Water is used as therapy for the sick as well as for those who are not ill. It is used to boost the immune system. This is hydrotherapy and there are many different forms. There is hydrotherapy that you can use if you are feeling sick such as standing in the bath, allow the hot water not boiling hit your back for approximately two minutes, and then turn the water to cold as much as you can stand, for approximately twenty-seconds. Do this about three times, always ending with cold water. Dry off and go to bed. It will make you feel sleepy. Do not get into your vehicle and drive you may fall asleep.

Salt glow bath is very good for circulation, removing dead skin as well as removing toxins from the body. You may use table salt, or Epson salt. Get a container, add Epson salt or combine with table salt, add a small amount of water to moisten the salt, run water over body, rub into the body, then wash off with cool water. This will do wonders for the body.

Chapter 5

Sleep

Sleep Deprivation And Mental Illness

It is very important to get a good night's sleep and there are consequences when you violate this vital part of not getting sleep the body so desperately needs to repair itself which is a part of the laws on healthy living.

Sleep is one of the most important laws of good health. If you are not getting enough sleep each night your body and your mind will soon break down and diseases will soon set in.

When your immune system becomes compromised due to sleeplessness, it leaves you susceptible in picking up various forms of diseases, which can be detrimental to your health.

Sometimes when you suffer from sleep insomnia you may stop feeling sleepy, or will want to sleep but is not able to do so, which can often times manifest itself as mental illness such as schizophrenia, dementia, nervousness, irritability, sudden rages, panic attacks, and hysteria

Not getting enough sleep can do a lot of harm to the human body and the brain which can also lead to deep or severe depression where the brain becomes compromised which causes emotional stress, psychological stress leading to hallucinations, nervousness, irritability, anxiety, psychotic behavior and not being able to function at your peek. These manifestations may not necessarily be mental illnesses but symptoms brought on by lack of sleep. Lack of sleep can affect your immune system and will lead to all kinds of illnesses and diseases.

Unfortunately, many doctors do not understand what is going on with the patient, and will prescribe long-term use of dangerous medication to take care of the problem. If the person goes several days and nights without sleep, then prescribing a medication to help the patient fall asleep will be needed at a low dosage.

If I were the patient or a member of the patient's family, this is what I would do; I would seek out natural forms of sleep aid and rid my body of dependency of prescription sleep aid. A good form of sleep aid is a product called Slumber, which is made up of herbs, such as Valerian root. This will not destroy the internal organs.

I would work with my doctor or health practitioner in helping with my sleep problem. I would try to fall asleep on my own after taking the natural herbs, and if I were still having some issue, would continue the use of it until I am able to develop a sleep pattern and fall asleep on my own.

I would go on a change of lifestyle using a vegetarian, preferable vegan diet. I would be careful what I watched, the music I listen to, the things I read, and the games I play. Remember that Satan seeks to destroy the mind. I would check my progesterone levels to see where they are, because sometimes the progesterone level is low, which can lead to lack of sleep. I would set a schedule for bedtime and do my best to stick to the schedule.

Please note: I am not a doctor or a health practitioner so I cannot give you advice on how to handle your mental health issue.

The Need For Getting Enough Sleep And Rest

We could learn a lot from the animals around us even when it comes to the importance of sleep and rest. We need to sleep and rest because it is important to our health and our well-being.

The bible states that Genesis 2:2 "And on the seventh day God ended his work which he had made; and he rested on the seventh day from all his work which he had made. " Genesis 2:3 Genesis 2:2, 3.

God was not tired when he rested but he rested to set an example for us to follow because He knows that not getting a good night rest would cause stress and sleep problems for the human race.

The seventh day was also a memorial of God creating the world. He set it aside for holy use. Jesus said to his disciples "Come ye yourselves apart into a desert place, and rest a while: for there were many coming and going, and they had no leisure so much as to eat." Mark 6:31.

Jesus saw that his disciples were exhausted from all the crowds that were following them, the disciples being of service to the people, were tired, and they were not getting enough rest that their bodies needed.

Jesus knew that it would not be good for their mental health would cause sleep problems and that would not be good for the disciples. It is hard to function due to lack of sleep and many accidents even fatal ones have been caused by drivers who fall asleep at the wheel while driving, so you can see that getting a good night's sleep in important to the body and to the mind.

Good Sleep For Good Health:

You need a good night sleep for good health and when you awake you are refreshed and ready for the challenges which lays ahead for that day.

When you get a good night sleep it gets rid of emotional stress, psychological stress, mental stress, cuts down on weight gain, headaches, chronic fatigue syndrome, and heart disease.

Getting a good nights sheep helps to regulate blood sugar, lower rates of death, diabetes, being able to concentrate better, to think better, rebuilds the tissues in the brain that has been damaged, repair the body and other health related benefits.

"When thou liest down, thou shalt not be afraid: yea, thou shalt lie down, and thy sleep shall be sweet." Proverbs 3:24.

Tips For Getting Better Sleep

Here are a few tips for getting better sleep. Avoid caffeine products, cigarettes, cigars, alcohol and all stimulants, set a bedtime schedule and stick to it. If at first you do not succeed, try and try and keep trying repeatedly. The body repairs itself between the hours of 9:00 p.m. and 12:00 midnight so try to set your bedtime between those hours as early as 9:00 p.m. to get the good quality sleep that your body needs.

We have been taught that we need at least eight to nine hours of sleep per night in order to promote good health. Your nightclothes should not be tight fitting and should be comfortable. For women, a bra or other restrictive article of clothing should not be worn to bed. You need to maintain good blood circulation.

Keep the sleeping area and bedroom as dark as possible and free from clutter which will help you to sleep better giving you a good night's rest. Sleeping better depends on you not using your bedroom or sleeping area as an office so remove the computers, the television, the stereo and other electronic devices and do not eat in the bedroom.

If you desire a good night, sleep keep the temperature in the room cool because if the room is hot it makes it very hard to sleep. If you are having problems falling asleep, try to relax because the mind sometimes refuses to shut itself down and is wired up. The mind will take you into areas that keeps you awake so try to think of the ocean, picture the waves going in and out and listen to the wind in your mind.

Getting deep sleep is important so purchase an air purifier, get a fan and turn them on. The air purifier and the fan will give off calm relaxing constant sounds to listen to, so try to concentrate on those sounds.

What kind of mattress are you sleeping on? If your mattress is in poor condition then it will affect the quality of your sleep. What about the pillow you sleep on, is it comfortable and well placed on the bed for optimum comfort?

Having good air quality in the bedroom is very important because if the air quality is poor this will affect not only your sleep but also your entire health.

Take deep breaths and listen to yourself as you breathe in and out; this may help you fall asleep. When your mind tries to take, you into one direction bring it back to the sound of the fan. You can also purchase a recording of the ocean or any other sounds that will be calming.

Try listening to soft music that is on a timer that will shut itself off after a pre-programmed amount of time that will allow you to fall asleep. This device can be kept on the outside of the bedroom but close enough so that you can hear it but not loud, where it will keep other members of your family awake.

To avoid getting up and going to the bathroom after you fall asleep try not to drink any liquid at least an hour and a half before bedtime which will contribute to lack of sleep.

Do not watch TV right before going to bed, take a warm relaxing bath and add some Epson salt to the water will help you to relax. Another problem is that maybe your magnesium level and your B vitamin levels may be low. Try adding some magnesium with B-6 and calcium along with some B-complex, which will benefit the body along with a good multivitamin.

Try not to resort to sleeping pills because you will become addicted to them and other side effects will be exhibited causing more problems. You could try using natural sleep aids such as herbs such as Valerian Root, Hops Strobile, Passionflower, Skullcap Aerial and other herbs to help you fall sleep, but don't feed on them.

There is a natural sleep aid product called "Slumber" that is also effective in helping those who need a little help in falling asleep and helping with some sleep disorder such as sleep insomnia. A cup of Chamomile tea and mint tea could be quite helpful.

If you are taking medications, please check with your doctor to make sure that none of the herbs you take will be a problem for you. In fact, before taking any herbal supplements always check with your doctor or health practitioner first and be very careful.

You may find other methods of falling asleep that may work for you, but remember, consistency is very important in anything that you do. If all else fail, get professional help from your doctor, or health care professional. Do not wait until mental symptoms appear, or the doctors will have you taking dangerous medications for the rest of your life, which you may not need.

Chapter 6

Sunlight

Can We Live Without Sunlight?

The earth cannot exist long term without sunlight. If the sun ceases to shine ever again all life forms on planet earth would cease to exist. That is how important sunlight is to all living things on earth. Sunlight is needed to regenerate the body, the animals, the plants and all living things. Our very existence depends on the sun.

Without sunlight the plants would die. The plants need sunlight in order to grow. Without sunlight, the animals would die so they also need the benefits of sunlight. Without sunlight all human beings on planet earth would die. Without sunlight every living thing in the sea, in the waters and on the earth would die. Sunlight is very important to life on planet earth. In other words, we must have sunlight if we are to live a healthy life.

The greater light that God made is the sun. "And God made the greater light to rule the day..." Genesis 1:16.

Benefits Of Sunlight

Sunlight stops depression, sunlight removes bacteria from the body and sunlight makes us well when we are sick. Sunlight is one of the laws of health that we should pay close attention to and we should not take for granted its benefits.

When a person is ill they should not be shut away from the sunlight because the sun has the ability to speed healing. The room where the sick person is should be well ventilated. The windows should be opened to allow adequate amount of sunlight to enter into the room and this will do wonders for the person who is sick. Turn off the air conditioner for a while and let the sunlight in to allow the patient to recover faster.

If the person is not too ill, take the patient outside into the sunlight during the early morning hours when it is not hot, and the sunlight will do wonders for that sick person. A person does not necessarily need to be in direct sunlight to reap the benefits of the sunlight.

Through sunlight, we get energy that is needed by the body, which helps our skin become radiant and healthy looking.

Sunlight A Natural Killer

Sunlight kills bacteria, germs, fungus, viruses and other organisms that invade our bodies and our homes. Staying in the sun for long periods is not advised due to the possibility of getting skin cancer.

Anyone having poor digestion can benefit from the sun. Getting sunlight will help with digestion by stimulating your digestive system and getting it to function the way it was made to function. A great way of increasing the white blood cells is to get a healthy dose of sunlight each day.

Try to get your sunlight during the early morning and later in the evening.

Vitamin D A Benefit Of Sunlight

Anyone who is deficient in vitamin D may want to spend more time exposed to sunlight. Exposure to sunlight can greatly boost the vitamin D level, which is beneficial in helping with the proper formation of the bones.

Sunlight helps the bones become strong and sunlight helps the bodies to fight against osteoporosis. Sunlight also has a direct benefit in boosting the immune system.

There is a better world to come where there will be no sickness, no one will need doctors. The Lord promises those who put their faith in him, believe his words, obey his commandments, including his health laws and accept him, as their personal savior will one day inherit eternal life.

This earth is not your home, you will live in heaven for a thousand years, then Jesus will recreate this earth as he did from the beginning, and you will see how he did it. It will be a marvelous day for all the

Redeemed. Now is the time to accept the Lord as your personal Savior, to give up a life of sin and follow the Lord wherever he leads.

This is what John the Revelator saw in vision as the Lord gave him a glimpse into heaven to give you hope for the future.

"And there shall in no wise enter into it any thing that defileth, neither whatsoever worketh abomination, or maketh a lie: but they which are written in the Lamb's book of life. And he shewed me a pure river of water of life, clear as crystal, proceeding out of the throne of God and of the Lamb.

In the midst of the street of it, and on either side of the river, was there the tree of life, which bare twelve manner of fruits, and yielded her fruit every month: and the leaves of the tree were for the healing of the nations." Revelation 21:27; 22: 1, 2.

www.ingramcontent.com/pod-product-compliance
Lightning Source LLC
Chambersburg PA
CBHW050503290526
45786CB00006B/2408